Contents

INTRODUCTION 2

What Is Cytotec? 3

What Are Side Effects of Cytotec? 3

Cytotec During Pregnancy and Breastfeeding 5

DESCRIPTION 10

Before Using 11

Indications & Dosage 13

Side Effects 24

Drug Interactions 32

Other Medical Problems 34

PRECAUTIONS 37

Special Note For Women 40

Pregnancy 42

Labor And Delivery 44

Nursing Mothers 48

OVERDOSE 49

CONTRAINDICATIONS 50

Storage 70

INTRODUCTION

Misoprostol is a synthetic prostaglandin E1 analogue that is used off-label for a variety of indications in the practice of obstetrics and gynecology, including medication abortion, medical management of miscarriage, induction of labor, cervical ripening before surgical procedures, and the treatment of postpartum hemorrhage. Due to its wide-ranging applications in reproductive health, misoprostol is on the World Health Organization Model List of Essential Medicines. This book briefly reviews the varied uses of misoprostol in obstetrics and gynecology.

What Is Cytotec?

Cytotec (misoprostol) is a synthetic (man-made) prostaglandin used to prevent the formation of ulcers in the stomach during treatment with aspirin or non-steroidal anti-inflammatory drugs (NSAIDs). NSAIDs and aspirin are used to treat pain, fever, arthritis, and inflammatory conditions. Cytotec is available in generic form.

What Are Side Effects of Cytotec?

Common side effects of Cytotec include:

diarrhea,

nausea,

vomiting,

stomach cramps,

gas,

constipation,

headache,

menstrual cramps,

spotting, or

increased or irregular menstruation.

Dosage for Cytotec

The recommended adult oral dose of Cytotec for

reducing the risk of NSAID-induced gastric ulcers

is 200 mcg four times daily with food.

What Drugs, Substances, or Supplements Interact with Cytotec?

Cytotec may interact with antacids that contain magnesium. Other drugs may also interact with Cytotec. Tell your doctor all prescription and over-the-counter medications and supplements you use.

Cytotec During Pregnancy and Breastfeeding
Cytotec must not be used during pregnancy to prevent stomach ulcers because of possible harm to a fetus. Use birth control while taking Cytotec and for at least one month or one completed menstrual cycle after you stop taking it. This medication passes into breast milk. This drug is

unlikely to harm a nursing infant. Consult your

doctor before breastfeeding.

Additional Information

Our Cytotec (misoprostol) Side Effects Drug

Center provides a comprehensive view of

available drug information on the potential side

effects when taking this medication.

WARNING

CYTOTEC (MISOPROSTOL) ADMINISTRATION TO

WOMEN WHO ARE PREGNANT CAN CAUSE BIRTH

DEFECTS, ABORTION, PREMATURE BIRTH OR
UTERINE RUPTURE.

UTERINE RUPTURE HAS BEEN REPORTED WHEN
CYTOTEC WAS ADMINISTERED IN PREGNANT
WOMEN TO INDUCE LABOR OR TO INDUCE
ABORTION. THE RISK OF UTERINE RUPTURE
INCREASES WITH ADVANCING GESTATIONAL
AGES AND WITH PRIOR UTERINE SURGERY,
INCLUDING CESAREAN DELIVERY (see also
PRECAUTIONS and Labor And Delivery).

CYTOTEC SHOULD NOT BE TAKEN BY PREGNANT
WOMEN TO REDUCE THE RISK OF ULCERS

INDUCED BY NONSTEROIDAL ANTI-

INFLAMMATORY DRUGS (NSAIDs) (see

CONTRAINDICATIONS, WARNINGS, and

PRECAUTIONS).

PATIENTS MUST BE ADVISED OF THE

ABORTIFACIENT PROPERTY AND WARNED NOT

TO GIVE THE DRUG TO OTHERS.

Cytotec should not be used for reducing the risk

of NSAID-induced ulcers in women of

childbearing potential unless the patient is at

high risk of complications from gastric ulcers

associated with use of the NSAID, or is at high

risk of developing gastric ulceration. In such

patients, Cytotec may be prescribed if the patient

has had a negative serum pregnancy test within 2 weeks prior to beginning therapy.

is capable of complying with effective contraceptive measures.

has received both oral and written warnings of the hazards of misoprostol, the risk of possible contraception failure, and the danger to other women of childbearing potential should the drug be taken by mistake.

will begin Cytotec only on the second or third day of the next normal menstrual period.

DESCRIPTION

Cytotec oral tablets contain either 100 mcg or 200 mcg of misoprostol, a synthetic prostaglandin E1 analog.

Misoprostol contains approximately equal amounts of the two diastereomers presented below with their enantiomers indicated by (±):

Cytotec® (misoprostol) - Structural Formula - Illustration

Misoprostol is a water-soluble, viscous liquid.

Inactive ingredients of tablets are hydrogenated castor oil, hypromellose, microcrystalline cellulose, and sodium starch glycolate.

Before Using

In deciding to use a medicine, the risks of taking the medicine must be weighed against the good it will do. This is a decision you and your doctor will make. For this medicine, the following should be considered:

Allergies

Tell your doctor if you have ever had any unusual or allergic reaction to this medicine or any other medicines. Also tell your health care professional if you have any other types of allergies, such as to foods, dyes, preservatives, or animals. For non-prescription products, read the label or package ingredients carefully.

Pediatric

Appropriate studies have not been performed on
the relationship of age to the effects of
misoprostol in the pediatric population. Safety
and efficacy have not been established.

Geriatric

Appropriate studies performed to date have not
demonstrated geriatric-specific problems that
would limit the usefulness of misoprostol in the
elderly.

Breastfeeding

There are no adequate studies in women for determining infant risk when using this medication during breastfeeding. Weigh the potential benefits against the potential risks before taking this medication while breastfeeding.

Indications & Dosage
INDICATIONS

Cytotec (misoprostol) is indicated for reducing the risk of NSAID (nonsteroidal anti-inflammatory drugs, including aspirin)–induced gastric ulcers in patients at high risk of complications from gastric ulcer, e.g., the elderly and patients with concomitant debilitating disease, as well as patients at high risk of developing gastric ulceration, such as patients with a history of ulcer. Cytotec has not been shown to reduce the risk of duodenal ulcers in patients taking NSAIDs. Cytotec should be taken for the duration of NSAID therapy. Cytotec has been shown to reduce the risk of gastric ulcers in controlled studies of 3 months' duration. It had no effect, compared to placebo, on gastrointestinal pain or discomfort associated with NSAID use.

DOSAGE AND ADMINISTRATION

The recommended adult oral dose of Cytotec for reducing the risk of NSAID-induced gastric ulcers is 200 mcg four times daily with food. If this dose cannot be tolerated, a dose of 100 mcg can be used. (See Clinical Studies.) Cytotec should be taken for the duration of NSAID therapy as prescribed by the physician. Cytotec should be taken with a meal, and the last dose of the day should be at bedtime.

Renal Impairment

Adjustment of the dosing schedule in renally impaired patients is not routinely needed, but dosage can be reduced if the 200-mcg dose is not tolerated. (See CLINICAL PHARMACOLOGY.)

SIDE EFFECTS

The following have been reported as adverse events in subjects receiving Cytotec:

Gastrointestinal

In subjects receiving Cytotec 400 or 800 mcg daily in clinical trials, the most frequent gastrointestinal adverse events were diarrhea and abdominal pain. The incidence of diarrhea at 800 mcg in controlled trials in patients on NSAIDs ranged from 14-40% and in all studies (over 5,000 patients) averaged 13%. Abdominal pain occurred in 13-20% of patients in NSAID trials and about 7% in all studies, but there was no consistent difference from placebo.

Diarrhea was dose related and usually developed early in the course of therapy (after 13 days), usually was self-limiting (often resolving after 8 days), but sometimes required discontinuation of Cytotec (2% of the patients). Rare instances of profound diarrhea leading to severe dehydration have been reported. Patients with an underlying condition such as inflammatory bowel disease, or those in whom dehydration, were it to occur, would be dangerous, should be monitored carefully if Cytotec is prescribed. The incidence of diarrhea can be minimized by administering after meals and at bedtime, and by avoiding coadministration of Cytotec with magnesium-containing antacids.

Gynecological

Women who received Cytotec during clinical trials reported the following gynecological disorders: spotting (0.7%), cramps (0.6%), hypermenorrhea (0.5%), menstrual disorder (0.3%) and dysmenorrhea (0.1%). Postmenopausal vaginal bleeding may be related to Cytotec administration. If it occurs, diagnostic workup should be undertaken to rule out gynecological pathology. (See BOXED WARNINGS.)

Elderly

There were no significant differences in the safety profile of Cytotec in approximately 500 ulcer patients who were 65 years of age or older compared with younger patients.

Additional adverse events which were reported are categorized as follows:

Incidence Greater Than 1%

In clinical trials, the following adverse reactions were reported by more than 1% of the subjects receiving Cytotec and may be causally related to the drug: nausea (3.2%), flatulence (2.9%),

headache (2.4%), dyspepsia (2.0%), vomiting

(1.3%), and constipation (1.1%). However, there

were no significant differences between the

incidences of these events for Cytotec and

placebo.

Causal Relationship Unknown

The following adverse events were infrequently

reported. Causal relationships between Cytotec

and these events have not been established but

cannot be excluded:

Body as a whole: aches/pains, asthenia, fatigue, fever, chills, rigors, weight changes.

Skin: rash, dermatitis, alopecia, pallor, breast pain.

Special senses: abnormal taste, abnormal vision, conjunctivitis, deafness, tinnitus, earache.

Respiratory: upper respiratory tract infection, bronchitis, bronchospasm, dyspnea, pneumonia, epistaxis.

Cardiovascular: chest pain, edema, diaphoresis, hypotension, hypertension, arrhythmia, phlebitis, increased cardiac enzymes, syncope, myocardial infarction (some fatal), thromboembolic events (e.g., pulmonary embolism, arterial thrombosis, and CVA).

Gastrointestinal: GI bleeding, GI inflammation/infection, rectal disorder, abnormal hepatobiliary function, gingivitis, reflux, dysphagia, amylase increase.

Hypersensitivity: anaphylactic reaction

Metabolic: glycosuria, gout, increased nitrogen, increased alkaline phosphatase.

Genitourinary: polyuria, dysuria, hematuria, urinary tract infection.

Nervous system/Psychiatric: anxiety, change in appetite, depression, drowsiness, dizziness, thirst, impotence, loss of libido, sweating

increase, neuropathy, neurosis, confusion.

Musculoskeletal: arthralgia, myalgia, muscle

cramps, stiffness, back pain.

Blood/Coagulation: anemia, abnormal

differential, thrombocytopenia, purpura, ESR

increased.

Along with its needed effects, a medicine may

cause some unwanted effects. Although not all of

these side effects may occur, if they do occur

they may need medical attention.

Side Effects

Check with your doctor immediately if any of the

following side effects occur:

Rare

Cramps

heavy bleeding

painful menstruation

Incidence not known

Bladder pain

bloody nose

bloody or black, tarry stools

bloody or cloudy urine

blurred vision

body aches or pain

chest pain

chills

confusion

constipation

cough

difficult, burning, or painful urination

difficulty with breathing

difficulty with moving

difficulty with swallowing

dizziness

dizziness, faintness, or lightheadedness when getting up suddenly from a lying or sitting position

ear congestion

feeling unusually cold

fever

frequent urge to urinate

headache

hives, itching, or skin rash

loss of voice

lower back or side pain

muscle pain or stiffness

nasal congestion

nervousness

pain in the joints

pale skin

pounding in the ears

puffiness or swelling of the eyelids or around the
eyes, face, lips, or tongue

runny nose

severe stomach pain

shivering

slow or fast heartbeat

sneezing

sore throat

sweating

tightness in the chest

troubled breathing with exertion

unusual bleeding or bruising

unusual tiredness or weakness

vomiting of blood or material that looks like coffee grounds

Some side effects may occur that usually do not need medical attention. These side effects may go away during treatment as your body adjusts to the medicine. Also, your health care professional may be able to tell you about ways to prevent or reduce some of these side effects. Check with your health care professional if any of the following side effects continue or are

bothersome or if you have any questions about

them:

More common

Abdominal or stomach pain

diarrhea

Less common

Acid or sour stomach

belching

bloated

excess air or gas in the stomach or intestines

full feeling

heartburn

indigestion

passing gas

stomach discomfort or upset

Incidence not known

Blistering, crusting, irritation, itching, or
reddening of the skin

breast pain

burning, dry, or itching eyes

change in taste

continuing ringing or buzzing or other
unexplained noise in the ears

cracked, dry, scaly skin

depression

discharge, excessive tearing

hair loss or thinning of the hair

hearing loss

lack or loss of strength

paleness of the skin

redness, pain, swelling of the eye, eyelid, or inner
lining of the eyelid

weight changes

Other side effects not listed may also occur in
some patients. If you notice any other effects,
check with your healthcare professional.

Call your doctor for medical advice about side effects. You may report side effects to the FDA at 1-800-FDA-1088.

Drug Interactions

Although certain medicines should not be used together at all, in other cases two different medicines may be used together even if an interaction might occur. In these cases, your doctor may want to change the dose, or other precautions may be necessary. When you are taking this medicine, it is especially important that your healthcare professional know if you are taking any of the medicines listed below. The following interactions have been selected on the basis of their potential significance and are not necessarily all-inclusive.

Using this medicine with any of the following medicines may cause an increased risk of certain side effects, but using both drugs may be the best treatment for you. If both medicines are prescribed together, your doctor may change the dose or how often you use one or both of the medicines.

Phenylbutazone

Other Interactions

Certain medicines should not be used at or around the time of eating food or eating certain types of food since interactions may occur. Using

alcohol or tobacco with certain medicines may

also cause interactions to occur. Discuss with

your healthcare professional the use of your

medicine with food, alcohol, or tobacco.

Other Medical Problems

The presence of other medical problems may

affect the use of this medicine. Make sure you

tell your doctor if you have any other medical

problems, especially:

Dehydration or

Heart or blood vessel problems or

Inflammatory bowel disease or

Stomach ulcers, history of—Use with caution.
May make these conditions worse.

Kidney disease—Use with caution. The effects
may be increased because of the slower removal
of the medicine from the body.

Proper Use

For safe and effective use of this medicine, do
not take more of it, do not take it more often,
and do not take it for a longer time than ordered
by your doctor. Taking too much of this medicine
may increase the chance of unwanted effects. Do
not change the dose or stop using this medicine
without checking first with your doctor.

This medicine should come with a patient information leaflet. Read and follow these instructions carefully. Ask your doctor if you have any questions.

Misoprostol is best taken with or after meals and at bedtime, unless otherwise directed by your doctor. To help prevent loose stools, diarrhea, and abdominal cramping, always take this medicine with food or milk.

Do not give this medicine to another person.

WARNINGS

See BOXED WARNINGS.

For hospital use only if misoprostol were to be used for cervical ripening, induction of labor, or for the treatment of serious post-partum hemorrhage, which are outside of the approved indication.

PRECAUTIONS

Caution should be employed when administering Cytotec (misoprostol) to patients with pre-existing cardiovascular disease.

Information For Patients

Women of childbearing potential using Cytotec to decrease the risk of NSAID-induced ulcers should be told that they must not be pregnant when Cytotec therapy is initiated, and that they must use an effective contraception method while taking Cytotec.

Cytotec is intended for administration along with nonsteroidal anti-inflammatory drugs (NSAIDs), including aspirin, to decrease the chance of developing an NSAID-induced gastric ulcer.

Cytotec should be taken only according to the directions given by a physician.

If the patient has questions about or problems with Cytotec, the physician should be contacted promptly.

THE PATIENT SHOULD NOT GIVE CYTOTEC TO ANYONE ELSE. Cytotec has been prescribed for the patient's specific condition, may not be the correct treatment for another person, and may be dangerous to the other person if she were to become pregnant.

The Cytotec package the patient receives from the pharmacist will include a leaflet containing patient information. The patient should read the leaflet before taking Cytotec and each time the prescription is renewed because the leaflet may have been revised.

Keep Cytotec out of the reach of children.

Special Note For Women

Cytotec may cause birth defects, abortion (sometimes incomplete), premature labor or rupture of the uterus if given to pregnant women.

Cytotec is available only as a unit-of-use package that includes a leaflet containing patient information. See PATIENT INFORMATION at the end of this labeling.

Carcinogenesis, Mutagenesis, Impairment Of Fertility

There was no evidence of an effect of Cytotec on tumor occurrence or incidence in rats receiving daily doses up to 150 times the human dose for 24 months. Similarly, there was no effect of Cytotec on tumor occurrence or incidence in mice receiving daily doses up to 1000 times the human dose for 21 months. The mutagenic potential of Cytotec was tested in several in vitro assays, all of which were negative.

Misoprostol, when administered to breeding male and female rats at doses 6.25 times to 625 times the maximum recommended human therapeutic dose, produced dose-related pre-and post-implantation losses and a significant

decrease in the number of live pups born at the

highest dose. These findings suggest the

possibility of a general adverse effect on fertility

in males and females.

Pregnancy
Teratogenic Effects

See BOXED WARNINGS. Congenital anomalies

sometimes associated with fetal death have been

reported subsequent to the unsuccessful use of

misoprostol as an abortifacient, but the drug's

teratogenic mechanism has not been

demonstrated. Several reports in the literature

associate the use of misoprostol during the first

trimester of pregnancy with skull defects, cranial nerve palsies, facial malformations, and limb defects.

Cytotec is not fetotoxic or teratogenic in rats and rabbits at doses 625 and 63 times the human dose, respectively.

Nonteratogenic Effects

See BOXED WARNINGS. Cytotec may endanger pregnancy (may cause abortion) and thereby cause harm to the fetus when administered to a pregnant woman. Cytotec may produce uterine contractions, uterine bleeding, and expulsion of the products of conception. Abortions caused by

Cytotec may be incomplete. If a woman is or becomes pregnant while taking this drug to reduce the risk of NSAID-induced ulcers, the drug should be discontinued and the patient apprised of the potential hazard to the fetus.

Labor And Delivery

Cytotec can induce or augment uterine contractions. Vaginal administration of Cytotec, outside of its approved indication, has been used as a cervical ripening agent, for the induction of labor and for treatment of serious postpartum hemorrhage in the presence of uterine atony. A major adverse effect of the obstetrical use of Cytotec is uterine tachysystole which may progress to uterine tetany with marked impairment of uteroplacental blood flow, uterine rupture (requiring surgical repair, hysterectomy, and/or salpingo-oophorectomy), or amniotic fluid embolism and lead to adverse fetal heart changes. Uterine activity and fetal status should be monitored by trained obstetrical personnel in a hospital setting.

The risk of uterine rupture associated with misoprostol use in pregnancy increases with advancing gestational ages and prior uterine surgery, including Cesarean delivery. Grand multiparity also appears to be a risk factor for uterine rupture.

The use of Cytotec outside of its approved indication may also be associated with meconium passage, meconium staining of amniotic fluid, and Cesarean delivery. Maternal shock, maternal death, fetal bradycardia, and fetal death have also been reported with the use of misoprostol.

Cytotec should not be used in the third trimester in women with a history of Cesarean section or major uterine surgery because of an increased risk of uterine rupture. Cytotec should not be used in cases where uterotonic drugs are generally contraindicated or where hyperstimulation of the uterus is considered inappropriate, such as cephalopelvic disproportion, grand multiparity, hypertonic or

hyperactive uterine patterns, or fetal distress

where delivery is not imminent, or when surgical

intervention is more appropriate.

The effect of Cytotec on later growth,

development, and functional maturation of the

child when Cytotec is used for cervical ripening or

induction of labor has not been established.

Information on Cytotec's effect on the need for

forceps delivery or other intervention is

unknown.

The use of Cytotec (misoprostol) for the

management of postpartum hemorrhage has

been associated with reports of high fevers

(greater than 40 degrees Celsius or 104 degrees

Fahrenheit), accompanied by autonomic and

central nervous system effects, such as

tachycardia, disorientation, agitation, and

convulsions. These fevers were transient in

nature. Supportive therapy should be dictated by

the patient's clinical presentation.

Nursing Mothers

Misoprostol is rapidly metabolized in the mother

to misoprostol acid, which is biologically active

and is excreted in breast milk. There are no

published reports of adverse effects of

misoprostol in breast-feeding infants of mothers

taking misoprostol. Caution should be exercised

when misoprostol is administered to a nursing

woman.

OVERDOSE

The toxic dose of Cytotec in humans has not

been determined. Cumulative total daily doses of

1600 mcg have been tolerated, with only

symptoms of gastrointestinal discomfort being

reported. In animals, the acute toxic effects are

diarrhea, gastrointestinal lesions, focal cardiac

necrosis, hepatic necrosis, renal tubular necrosis,

testicular atrophy, respiratory difficulties, and

depression of the central nervous system. Clinical

signs that may indicate an overdose are sedation,

tremor, convulsions, dyspnea, abdominal pain,

diarrhea, fever, palpitations, hypotension, or bradycardia. Symptoms should be treated with supportive therapy.

It is not known if misoprostol acid is dialyzable. However, because misoprostol is metabolized like a fatty acid, it is unlikely that dialysis would be appropriate treatment for overdosage.

CONTRAINDICATIONS

Cytotec should not be taken by pregnant women to reduce the risk of ulcers induced by nonsteroidal anti-inflammatory drugs (NSAIDs).

Cytotec should not be taken by anyone with a history of allergy to prostaglandins.

Clinical Pharmacology

CLINICAL PHARMACOLOGY

Pharmacokinetics

Misoprostol is extensively absorbed, and

undergoes rapid de-esterification to its free acid,

which is responsible for its clinical activity and,

unlike the parent compound, is detectable in

plasma. The alpha side chain undergoes beta

oxidation and the beta side chain undergoes

omega oxidation followed by reduction of the

ketone to give prostaglandin F analogs.

In normal volunteers, Cytotec (misoprostol) is rapidly absorbed after oral administration with a Tmax of misoprostol acid of 12 ± 3 minutes and a terminal half-life of 20–40 minutes.

There is high variability of plasma levels of misoprostol acid between and within studies but mean values after single doses show a linear relationship with dose over the range of 200–400 mcg. No accumulation of misoprostol acid was noted in multiple dose studies; plasma steady state was achieved within two days.

Maximum plasma concentrations of misoprostol acid are diminished when the dose is taken with food and total availability of misoprostol acid is reduced by use of concomitant antacid. Clinical trials were conducted with concomitant antacid, however, so this effect does not appear to be clinically important

After oral administration of radiolabeled misoprostol, about 80% of detected radioactivity appears in urine. Pharmacokinetic studies in patients with varying degrees of renal impairment showed an approximate doubling of T½, Cmax, and AUC compared to normals, but no clear correlation between the degree of impairment and AUC. In subjects over 64 years of age, the AUC for misoprostol acid is increased. No routine dosage adjustment is recommended in older patients or patients with renal impairment, but dosage may need to be reduced if the usual dose is not tolerated.

Drug interaction studies between misoprostol and several nonsteroidal anti-inflammatory drugs showed no effect on the kinetics of ibuprofen or diclofenac, and a 20% decrease in aspirin AUC, not thought to be clinically significant.

Pharmacokinetic studies also showed a lack of drug interaction with antipyrine and propranolol when these drugs were given with misoprostol. Misoprostol given for 1 week had no effect on the steady state pharmacokinetics of diazepam when the two drugs were administered 2 hours apart.

The serum protein binding of misoprostol acid is less than 90% and is concentration-independent in the therapeutic range.

After a single oral dose of misoprostol to nursing mothers, misoprostol acid was excreted in breast milk. The maximum concentration of misoprostol acid in expressed breast milk was achieved within 1 hour after dosing and was 7.6 pg/ml (CV 37%) and 20.9 pg/ml (CV 62%) after single 200 µg and 600 µg misoprostol administration, respectively. The misoprostol acid concentrations in breast milk declined to < 1 pg/ml at 5 hours post-dose.

Pharmacodynamics

Misoprostol has both antisecretory (inhibiting gastric acid secretion) and (in animals) mucosal protective properties. NSAIDs inhibit prostaglandin synthesis, and a deficiency of prostaglandins within the gastric mucosa may lead to diminishing bicarbonate and mucus secretion and may contribute to the mucosal damage caused by these agents. Misoprostol can increase bicarbonate and mucus production, but in man this has been shown at doses 200 mcg and above that are also antisecretory. It is therefore not possible to tell whether the ability of misoprostol to reduce the risk of gastric ulcer is the result of its antisecretory effect, its

mucosal protective effect, or both.

In vitro studies on canine parietal cells using

tritiated misoprostol acid as the ligand have led

to the identification and characterization of

specific prostaglandin receptors. Receptor

binding is saturable, reversible, and

stereospecific. The sites have a high affinity for

misoprostol, for its acid metabolite, and for other

E type prostaglandins, but not for F or I

prostaglandins and other unrelated compounds,

such as histamine or cimetidine. Receptor-site

affinity for misoprostol correlates well with an

indirect index of antisecretory activity. It is likely

that these specific receptors allow misoprostol taken with food to be effective topically, despite the lower serum concentrations attained.

Misoprostol produces a moderate decrease in pepsin concentration during basal conditions, but not during histamine stimulation. It has no significant effect on fasting or postprandial gastrin nor on intrinsic factor output.

Effects On Gastric Acid Secretion

Misoprostol, over the range of 50–200 mcg, inhibits basal and nocturnal gastric acid secretion, and acid secretion in response to a variety of stimuli, including meals, histamine, pentagastrin, and coffee. Activity is apparent 30 minutes after oral administration and persists for at least 3 hours. In general, the effects of 50 mcg were modest and shorter lived, and only the 200-mcg dose had substantial effects on nocturnal secretion or on histamine and meal-stimulated secretion.

Uterine Effects

Cytotec has been shown to produce uterine contractions that may endanger pregnancy. (See BOXED WARNINGS.)

Other Pharmacologic Effects

Cytotec does not produce clinically significant effects on serum levels of prolactin, gonadotropins, thyroid-stimulating hormone, growth hormone, thyroxine, cortisol, gastrointestinal hormones (somatostatin, gastrin, vasoactive intestinal polypeptide, and motilin), creatinine, or uric acid. Gastric emptying, immunologic competence, platelet aggregation, pulmonary function, or the cardiovascular system are not modified by recommended doses of Cytotec.

Clinical Studies

In a series of small short-term (about 1 week) placebo-controlled studies in healthy human volunteers, doses of misoprostol were evaluated for their ability to reduce the risk of NSAID-induced mucosal injury. Studies of 200 mcg q.i.d. of misoprostol with tolmetin and naproxen, and of 100 and 200 mcg q.i.d. with ibuprofen, all showed reduction of the rate of significant endoscopic injury from about 70–75% on placebo to 10–30% on misoprostol. Doses of 25–200 mcg q.i.d. reduced aspirin-induced mucosal injury and bleeding.

Reducing The Risk Of Gastric Ulcers Caused By Nonsteroidal Anti-Inflammatory Drugs (NSAIDs)

Two 12-week, randomized, double-blind trials in osteoarthritic patients who had gastrointestinal symptoms but no ulcer on endoscopy while taking an NSAID compared the ability of 200 mcg of Cytotec, 100 mcg of Cytotec, and placebo to reduce the risk of gastric ulcer (GU) formation. Patients were approximately equally divided between ibuprofen, piroxicam, and naproxen, and continued this treatment throughout the 12 weeks. The 200-mcg dose caused a marked, statistically significant reduction in gastric ulcers in both studies. The lower dose was somewhat less effective, with a significant result in only one of the studies.

In these trials there were no significant differences between Cytotec and placebo in relief of day or night abdominal pain. No effect of

Cytotec in reducing the risk of duodenal ulcers was demonstrated, but relatively few duodenal lesions were seen.

In another clinical trial, 239 patients receiving aspirin 650–1300 mg q.i.d. for rheumatoid arthritis who had endoscopic evidence of duodenal and/or gastric inflammation were randomized to misoprostol 200 mcg q.i.d. or placebo for 8 weeks while continuing to receive aspirin. The study evaluated the possible interference of Cytotec on the efficacy of aspirin in these patients with rheumatoid arthritis by analyzing joint tenderness, joint swelling, physician's clinical assessment, patient's assessment, change in ARA classification, change in handgrip strength, change in duration of morning stiffness, patient's assessment of pain at rest, movement, interference with daily activity, and ESR. Cytotec did not interfere with the efficacy of aspirin in these patients with rheumatoid arthritis.

Animal Toxicology

A reversible increase in the number of normal surface gastric epithelial cells occurred in the dog, rat, and mouse. No such increase has been observed in humans administered Cytotec for up to 1 year.

An apparent response of the female mouse to Cytotec in long-term studies at 100 to 1000 times the human dose was hyperostosis, mainly of the medulla of sternebrae. Hyperostosis did not occur in long-term studies in the dog and rat and has not been seen in humans treated with Cytotec.

PATIENT INFORMATION

Read this leaflet before taking Cytotec® (misoprostol) and each time your prescription is renewed, because the leaflet may be changed.

Cytotec (misoprostol) is being prescribed by your doctor to decrease the chance of getting stomach ulcers related to the arthritis/pain medication that you take.

Do not take Cytotec to reduce the risk of NSAID-induced ulcers if you are pregnant. (See BOXED WARNINGS.) Cytotec can cause abortion (sometimes incomplete which could lead to dangerous bleeding and require hospitalization and surgery), premature birth, or birth defects. It is also important to avoid pregnancy while taking this medication and for at least one month or through one menstrual cycle after you stop taking it. Cytotec may cause the uterus to tear (uterine rupture) during pregnancy. The risk of uterine rupture increases as your pregnancy advances and if you have had surgery on the uterus, such as a Cesarean delivery. Rupture (tearing) of the uterus can result in severe bleeding, hysterectomy, and/or maternal or fetal death.

If you become pregnant during Cytotec therapy, stop taking Cytotec and contact your physician immediately. Remember that even if you are on a means of birth control it is still possible to become pregnant. Should this occur, stop taking Cytotec and contact your physician immediately.

Cytotec may cause diarrhea, abdominal cramping, and/or nausea in some people. In most cases these problems develop during the first few weeks of therapy and stop after about a week. You can minimize possible diarrhea by making sure you take Cytotec with food.

Because these side effects are usually mild to moderate and usually go away in a matter of days, most patients can continue to take Cytotec. If you have prolonged difficulty (more than 8 days), or if you have severe diarrhea, cramping and/or nausea, call your doctor.

Take Cytotec only according to the directions given by your physician.

Do not give Cytotec to anyone else. It has been prescribed for your specific condition, may not be the correct treatment for another person, and would be dangerous if the other person were pregnant.

This information sheet does not cover all possible side effects of Cytotec. This patient information leaflet does not address the side effects of your arthritis/pain medication. See your doctor if you have questions.

Keep out of reach of children.

Storage

Store the medicine in a closed container at room temperature, away from heat, moisture, and direct light. Keep from freezing.

Keep out of the reach of childre

Do not keep outdated medicine or medicine no longer needed.

Ask your healthcare professional how you should dispose of any medicine you do not use.

Made in the USA
Columbia, SC
17 September 2023

23002236R00039